GET THE REAL SKINNY ON GLUTEN-FREE LIVING

Simple Steps To Break Up With Gluten

BY ROXANNE N. MCDONALD

Published by Epic Health Now
Los Angeles, California

Roxanne McDonald

This book remains the copyrighted property of the author, and may not be reproduced, copied and distributed for commercial or non-commercial purposes. Thank you for your support.

Medical Disclaimer

This book contains general information about gluten, wheat, grains, dairy, and soy related medical conditions. This information is intended for informational purposes only and should not be considered medical advice from a licensed medical professional. The reader should regularly consult a Physician in matters relating to her/his health and particularly with respect to any symptoms that may require diagnosis or medical attention. The author and publisher specifically disclaim all responsibility for any liability, loss or risk, personal or otherwise, which is incurred as a consequence, directly or indirectly, from the use or application of any contents of this book. By reading beyond this disclaimer, each reader agrees the author may not be held responsible for any such consequences.

Roxanne McDonald

Trademark Disclaimer

Mention of any companies, organizations, or products in this book are the trademarks of their respective owners. It does not imply endorsement by the publisher, nor does reference to specific companies, organizations or products imply that they endorse this book.

Roxanne N. McDonald
Epic Health Now

Visit us on the Web:
http://www.epichealthnow.com
E-Mail: roxanne@epichealthnow.com

Dedicated to

Your Health

Roxanne McDonald

Contents

Desserts

Introduction

I am a writer, advocate for nutrition, spiritual practitioner, adventure seeker, and business person all wrapped up into one. After many years as an executive in Corporate America, I have been pulled to follow a path of healthy eating, being and doing.

Based on my own personal challenges with gluten, and having witnessed what it does to others, I chose this topic to become more aware of its effects. There are many adverse reactions these illusive protein strands cause.

The ultimate service is to pass this information on. My intention is to help enlighten others who may be suffering from, "not feeling good," without really knowing the cause. It is so important to recognize the myriad of choices we all have to create a magnificent life. It is equally empowering and significant to develop new patterns that will help to ensure sustainability. An open mind will take us to these places and beyond!

There is, without question, a shift that is taking place on a global level. Older paradigms are crumbling. Standards of food and diet are a part of this transformation. I think it's a great thing – albeit a bit scary and unfamiliar. The examination of the information given here is absolutely necessary in order for new ideas, and ways of being, to take root.

The medical, nutritional, psychological, naturopathic, physical therapeutic, and chiropractic professions are joining together with emphasis on addressing and treating the root cause of sickness. It is a powerful experience to be a part of, and it is going to happen no matter what. The Universe sets its course and does its thing. Let us all share in this EPIC transformation!

Chapter 1

That Gut Feeling: Can You and Gluten Agree to Disagree?

Question: What is one of the most addictive cravings people experience when eating food?

Answer: Texture. It may be firm or soft, crispy or spongy, smooth or crunchy; most of us fall in love with the way food "feels" in our mouth. This is where gluten arrives on the scene.

Gluten is used in the manufacturing of all packaged, boxed and canned processed

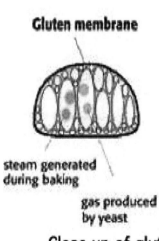 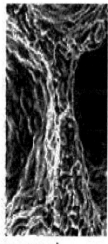 foods to create textures that are more palatabl e to our

Close up of gluten yeast

taste buds. It is also used to thicken, bind and coat. Gluten is even used as glue on envelopes and stamps! Scary, huh?

Gluten is a generic term for the storage proteins found in many grains. Wheat, flour products, bread, barley & rye, also white (refined) sugar, are some of the foods that contain specific amino acid sequences harmful to people. *Celiac Sprue*, the clinical term used for those afflicted by the consumption of foods that contain gluten, basically causes damage to the lining of the small intestine. This autoimmune condition leaves "self-attacking-self" as a misdirection of a faltering immune system.

The sad part about this disorder is that there are many people who are allergic to gluten and have no clue. I was one of them! It wasn't until I underwent a targeted muscle testing procedure, that I found out I was allergic to grains... wheat in particular. The symptoms can vary from person to person. One may be asymptomatic, not feeling anything, someone else may suffer from chronic digestive distress and there are others who experience constant fatigue. I know nowadays if I've eaten anything with gluten in it because the joints in my hands start screaming at me!

What are Signs of Gluten Intolerance?

Some of the symptoms to look for when dealing with the "gluten monster" are as follows:

- Iron deficiency anemia
- Bone or joint pain
- Arthritis
- Osteoporosis
- Depression or anxiety
- Tingling or numbness in hands and feet.
- Seizures
- Infertility or current miscarriage
- Canker sores inside the mouth
- Itchy skin rash

Other startling facts about Celiac disease are:

• One out of every 133 Americans has Celiac disease. 97% of Americans estimated to have CD are not diagnosed. 30% of the US population is estimated to have the genes necessary for Celiac disease.

• 2.5 babies are born every minute in the USA with the genetic makeup to have Celiac disease.

• Celiac disease affects more people in the US than Crohn's Disease, Cystic Fibrosis, Multiple Sclerosis and Parkinson's disease combined.

• Even though a simple blood test exists, it takes an average of 11 years for patients to be properly diagnosed with Celiac disease.

- 12% of people in the US who have Downs Syndrome also have Celiac disease.

- 6% of people in the US who have Type 1 Diabetes also have Celiac disease.

Historically Speaking

London physician Samuel Gee has been credited with being the first to describe Celiac disease in his famous article, "On the Coeliac Affection," published in the St. Bartholomew's Hospital Report in 1888. The word *coeliacus,* is Latin, which comes from the Greek word *koiliakos. Koilia* in Greek means abdomen. The microscopic, hair-like projections, (villi), in the small intestine provide the surface area needed to absorb the nutrients from the foods and supplements you ingest. When the gut becomes leaky, the food foregoes proper digestion.

The link between this disease and diet didn't take place until 1944, when a Dutch pediatrician noticed that the children from his clinic started getting better after the Nazi invasion. Previous symptoms of bloating, stomach cramping, diarrhea and fatigue gradually lessened, as bread disappeared from their diets, though these actions were punitive and the children were starving for food.

You may be asking right about now: How do I know if I'm a high risk for CD? Excellent question!

Various reports land causes anywhere from genetic predisposition to cultural tendencies; all of which are valid projections. However, at the end of the day the ultimate *healing* takes place with the elimination of gluten from the diet.

Nutritional studies reveal people eat foods that are unnatural for the body's digestive system. Our current society's temperament shows it to be especially true. Most of the food we have available to consume has been altered from its original source: the way nature made it. Biochemists have changed the seeds from which plants are grown, and food manufacturers have inundated our food supply with gluten, most notably wheat.

When people show up to nutritionists for help one of the first things examined is their diet for *questionable* foods. These include: milk, eggs, fish, crustacean shellfish, tree nuts, peanuts, wheat, soybeans, peppers, tomatoes, and eggplants.

Clients are then encouraged to modify their diets by eliminating irritating foods and their derivatives. Next, wholesome nutrition is introduced; which includes more organic plant based foods, as well as supplements to compensate for present deficiencies.

Not Oatmeal! Say it ain't so!

Needless to say, I experienced somewhat of a meltdown when I realized that I might have to...kick the oatmeal habit. The debate over whether there is gluten in oatmeal has been somewhat controversial for years. But all in all, the oats win! Historically, oats have not been included in gluten-free diets throughout the United States. However, recommendations on oat consumption are changing as a result of thorough, analytical studies conducted since 1995 that indicate that people allergic to gluten can safely eat moderate amounts of oats uncontaminated with wheat, barley, or rye.

Several studies have been performed investigating the safety of oats, using an intestinal biopsy as a method of investigation. The intestinal biopsy is considered the best available test for diagnosing Celiac disease. Participants of these studies were usually recently diagnosed with Celiac disease, or in remission.

The procedure typically entailed an intestinal biopsy before the start of the study, whereby the participants consumed daily amounts of oats for the length of the period. When they reached the end of the research term, they participated in another biopsy. Both before and after biopsies were compared, to determine whether oat consumption had either supported or interrupted recovery of the intestinal lining. These recent studies have concluded that moderate amounts of uncontaminated oats are safe for consumption by most people who are allergic to gluten.

Other studies have found a small group of participants to be negatively affected by oats; further research revealed that these patients were exposed to avenin – the gluten protein found in oats. When exposed in a test tube, researchers were able to identify lymphocytes: small white blood cells which play a significant role in defending the body's immune system, made specifically in response to avenin.

The researchers concluded that some persons with Celiac disease have lymphocytes in their intestinal lining which can react with particular oat protein and cause inflammation.

Bear in mind that the number of people harmed by oats, appears to be small. You may want to discuss with your physician or health care practitioner whether periodical allergenic testing could be helpful.

Roxanne McDonald

Chapter 2

My name is _____ and I'm a Gluten addict.

Do you ever have serious cravings for breads, pastas and other complex carbohydrates? I know I have. *And* I've had to admit to the addictions I've developed for certain foods.

The body reacts to foods where there is an allergic or intolerant response by producing its own addictive narcotic, the opioid endorphins. They create a feeling of euphoria when that particular food is consumed. You begin to crave these foods when you eat them because they induce a pleasurable response.

The relationship between food addiction, gluten intolerance, and alcoholism, is well documented. Gluten breaks down in the body as sugar, its consumption signals a *feel-good* endorphin reaction, and when ingested by gluten intolerant individuals that can induce serious binging.

Food addiction is not just a psychological dilemma of will power; there is a chemical imbalance as well. Food addicts suffer from altered brain chemistry. Their feel good transmitter, serotonin, may be at lower levels, or they may suffer from the effects of protein malabsorption, or an imbalanced metabolism. When people are low in serotonin, they crave carbohydrates like ice cream, or combinations of grains and dairy products, such as cereal and milk, often times in the evening hours.

Consumption of these foods temporarily raises the serotonin levels in the brain.

Dependency on food can cause compulsive overeating, anorexia, bulimia, obesity, and can bring on feelings of depression and anxiety. Food addiction is synonymous with chemical dependency, triggered by consumption. Avoiding these specific foods is the answer.

We *must* eliminate refined sugar; which is as powerful as heroin, white flour, processed foods, and caffeine (I know ouch!) and replace them with more nutrient-rich, organic, whole foods.

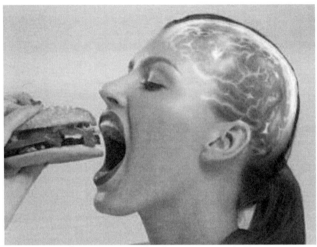

Food is intended to nourish, not nurture. Typically, from the moment of birth, we have been nurtured with food as the primary symbol of comfort. Our initial experience was our mother's milk, which we both nourished and nurtured. We must reprogram our relationship with food and choose the kinds of foods that nourish us, and offer the correct macronutrient proportions to our physiology. This will lead to maintaining blood sugar stability and eventually eliminating cravings.

Some Characteristics of Food Addiction

Food and alcohol addicts tend to suffer from hypoglycemia (low blood sugar); they can experience sweets and carbohydrates cravings, mood swings/irritability, alcohol cravings, gluten intolerance and adrenal fatigue. These symptoms can all be corrected by shifting your diet. This means eliminating gluten, dairy, soy, refined sugars and processed foods, and consuming plenty of nutrient rich vegetables, fruits and proteins from organic sources.

It is of vital importance for us to treat the cause, instead of the symptoms. Some questions to ask yourself regarding possible gluten intolerance and or food addictions are:

- What is your initial memory of food?
- Do you have a history of eating disorders and/or alcoholism in your family?
- What is your family's relationship with food?
- What is your relationship with food?
- Are you an obsessive over eater? Under eater?
- When was your first problem with food? What were the circumstances?
- Do you use drugs or alcohol to manipulate your weight?

- Are you or anyone else concerned about your eating habits or your weight?

- Is there anything you eat too little or too much of?

- How often are you eating?

These types of questions may be quite confrontational and bring up defensive resistance, at first. They can, nevertheless, most assuredly lead down a path where you can considerably change your overall health: physical, mental, nutritional and spiritual, for your greater good! We'll share more on how later on in the book.

Roxanne McDonald

Chapter 3

Foods That Surprisingly Contain Gluten

My quest to eat gluten-free has been quite a revealing experience.

A recent article from, *Everyday Health,* revealed that some of the hidden sources of gluten are often overlooked. Wheat-free items can also pose a threat if they contain other forms of gluten, like barley, or rye. Hence, scrutinize packaged food labels before you buy. I'll admit I've become that irritating patron who grills the waiter about every ingredient before ordering my food. It is necessary, so there are no menacing surprises after eating.

Interestingly enough, there are certain non-food items that contain various forms of hidden gluten. And while the Food and Drug Administration (FDA) has recently begun implementing gluten-free labeling standards for food products, these standards do not apply to every item that could contain gluten.

What Non-Food Products contain Gluten?

Some other sources to put on your radar that may contain gluten are:

• Medications – this one may come as a surprise to you. When you look at the word gluten, think *glue*. It is often used as a binder. The National Foundation for Celiac Awareness (NFCA) has successfully educated the public on this issue, which has led to efforts on part of the FDA to address medication labeling, which currently does not include specific mention of gluten or wheat products. It can be difficult to determine what medications have gluten in them or not, the NFCA indicates that generics seem more likely to have traces of gluten.

• Beauty Products - The 2011 annual meeting of the American College of Gastroenterology presented research demonstrating how difficult it is for consumers to find out if their beauty products contain any gluten. Though you are not actually eating your make-up, lip balm that has even a small amount of gluten could cause a problem. Think of how often you bite or lick your lips.

• Questions have been raised by researchers regarding whether gluten containing moisturizers and lotions may trigger a reaction in the skin of a person with Celiac disease. The investigation was a result of case studies of two women who had contact irritation on their skin that went away when they eliminated gluten from their diet and stopped using beauty products that contained gluten. Hydrolyzed, gluten in beauty products is used to help thicken and stabilize the product. This area is undergoing further research exploration. Basically, people with gluten intolerance, who want to live a gluten-free life style, should be aware of the ingredients in their cosmetics.

• Similar to prescription medication and cosmetics, gluten may appear in vitamin supplements purely as a binding agent, according to the NFCA.

Some Foods to be Aware of that Contain Gluten are:

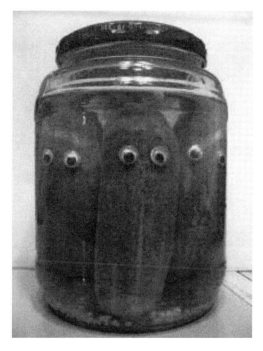

- Pickles: The problem with pickles is beer. Some pickling processes include malt vinegar (a beer-like liquid) which may contain gluten.

- Bouillon cubes: This seemingly harmless soup base can be a gluten cesspool. The ingredient to avoid is maltodextrin, a thickening based gluten product. What's better is if you take the time to make your own stock, and use it for soups and stews.

• Gravy: Gravies made from flour are obvious sources of gluten, and so are most instant gravy packets. You may use cornstarch at home as a thickener; away from home it may be best to stay off the gravy.

• Blue cheese: There are contradictory messages about these blue veined cheeses. Bread mold may be used to make them. Though the amount of gluten found in blue cheese may be considered to be a minute amount, gluten intolerant people may want to stay clear.

• Hot dogs: Yes, this beloved ballpark munchie could be loaded with gluten. Read the labels to find a brand without it.

- Soy sauce: Wheat in soy sauce? You may be asking. And yes, wheat is a key part of the manufacturing process, which makes the flavoring problematic for people with gluten intolerance. Try gluten-free tamari instead.

- Hot chocolate: How about those cold wintery nights when you invite in a hot cup of cocoa? You are going to want to make sure to read the ingredients of prepackaged cocoa mixes, which may be processed on machine exposed to wheat products and subject to gluten cross contamination. Consider making it from scratch with organic cacao, almond, or rice milk, coconut sugar, or organic cane sugars, or stevia – a natural plant based sweetener. Also, as a nice treat top it off with marshmallows; they are gluten-free!

- French fries: When eating out, especially fast-food restaurants, you also run the risk of cross – contamination. Though an order of French fries may initially be gluten-free, if they are fried in the same oil as onion rings or hush puppies: gluten-free no more! Check before you order.

Also bear in mind: Labels that read, *wheat free*, do not necessarily mean there is no gluten in the food. Other grains (such as barley and rye) take ownership of the difficult-to-digest protein strand as well.

It is highly recommended for you to visit your farmer's markets and whole food stores, master your food domain and prepare your own meals more often. You'll gain control over what you eat and how it tastes. Remember: read those labels!

Chapter 4

Other Diseases Hiding Behind Gluten

How daunting can it be when things begin to unravel and you find a disease within a disease?! Gluten intolerance (Celiac disease) is showing up in many other forms that are to be taken quite seriously as well.

Tired of Scratching that Itch?

One of the repercussions of gluten sensitivity is skin disorders. Ever had an itch that you just couldn't scratch enough?

A chronic itch recently recognized and accepted as a form of gluten insensitivity is *dermatitis herpetiformis*: DH. American dermatologist, Louis Duhring, first described DH within a clinical environment back in 1884. However, it wasn't until 1967 that it was actually connected to gluten intolerance.

DH shows up as small patches of red blisters often found on the back of the elbow and forearms, on the buttocks, and in front of the knees. This disease, though most notably found amongst young people, can affect anyone.

The immune system is reacting to ingested gluten, creating DH. The body, instead of digesting the protein strand, fights it with antibodies produced in the intestine. These antibodies collide with the gluten, ultimately causing blockages in the blood stream. The blockage incites the gathering of white blood cells to fight the invasion, and the white blood cells in turn, emit potent chemicals that cause the rash.

Though the gastric, stomach-plaguing symptoms typically found with gluten intolerance did not reveal themselves in this case, the debilitating condition was relieved once associated with gluten consumption, and a change of diet.

One person stricken with DH described it as feeling like, "hundreds of tiny swords were being jabbed into me, all at the same time." ☹

Imagine the suffering so many others have experienced due to misdiagnosis, because doctors didn't recognize it as an allergic reaction to gluten in foods!

There are other skin disorders such as psoriasis, dermatitis, eczema, rosacea, even severe acne that has been repeatedly shown to be directly related to eating habits. Recent studies continue to reveal that undiagnosed gluten allergies can be the cause of these previously mentioned skin diseases. Many documented cases reveal, when gluten is eliminated from the patients' diet, their skin ailment goes away.

Muscular Disorders

How's your muscular coordination these days? No, I'm not talking about being swift afoot with the latest dance moves. I'm referring to a loss of muscle control that may source back to something you ate.

Sporadic Ataxia, a fancier name for irregular loss of muscle coordination, currently has no known cause. People who have this condition show these symptoms:

- Problems with walking coordination
- Difficulty engaging motor skills
- Slurred speech
- Drooling
- Speedy, unfocused vision

This neurological disorder presently affects an estimated 300,000 Americans based on reports. Though doctors have yet to locate the root cause, one possibility frequently overlooked that needs to be considered is gluten sensitivity.

The University of Maryland study and *The Annals of Medicine* in 2010 stated that since 1974 the rate of autoimmune diseases such as rheumatoid arthritis, lupus and multiple sclerosis has doubled every 15 years and gluten is suspect.

Researchers found that the number of people with blood markers for Celiac disease has increased steadily from one in 501 in 1974; to one in 219 in 1989; to one in 133 in 2005; and now one in 98 as recent as 2011.

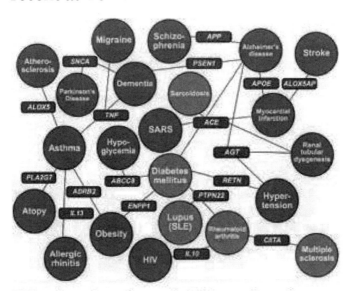

Blood markers (samples) for celiac disease

"You're never too old to develop gluten intolerance", states Alessio Fasano, M.D., director of the University of

Maryland's Mucosal Biology Research Center and the Celiac research center, which conducted the study.

The Universita Politecnica delle Marche in Ancona, Italy; the John Hopkins Bloomberg School of Public Health; the Women and Children's hospital of Buffalo; and Quest Diagnostics Inc. of San Juan Capistrano Ca., also participated.

The incidence of gluten intolerance rose, as people in the study aged. Findings reveal the disease can rear its ugly head in early childhood as well. Though researchers have identified definitive genetic markers for the development of Celiac disease, the medical field is still quite bewildered as to how and why an individual loses tolerance to gluten.

The bottom line continues to confirm that individuals who have maintained a gluten-free diet show a significant improvement in overall performance, showing dramatic improvement with their neurological tests results. The others who continued their same eating habits continued to get worse. The power of choice is a wonderful thing.

Headaches

A study was conducted in 2004, exploring the connection between gluten sensitivity and severe headaches. The focus centered on "soft" neurological conditions such as headaches in young adults and children. The most common neurological disorder found in the 111 patients tested was harsh headaches. Research findings revealed: 64.5% had late onset symptoms of gluten allergies, and 35.5% had the early infantile form of Celiac disease.

The breakdown regarding the types of headaches was:

- Migraine : 41.4%
- Non specific : 35.5%
- Tension-psychogenic: 19.4%

There was a study where sixteen volunteers were stricken with oppressive headaches: nine with migraines and seven with nonspecific. They were put on a gluten-free diet, and invariably all were relieved of their symptoms.

An earlier study, administered in 2001, chronicled 10 patients; all of whom were plagued with migraine headaches. Each had MRI testing, which indicated inflammation of the central nervous system, and each was found to be sensitive to gluten. It was recommended that these patients start a gluten-free diet.

All but one patient found relief. Seven of the ten experienced complete relief, while two had partial improvement. The one patient who continued to suffer from headaches, refused to try the gluten-free diet.

This next case illustrates the power of a gluten-free diet: A 50 year-old-man, who did not have a medical history of migraines, began to experience severe headaches which lasted for four years. His pain increased with such severity that he agreed to undergo a blood test. The test revealed he had anti-gliadin antibodies: an allergic reaction to wheat.

He began a gluten-free diet, and after a while his balance greatly improved, and his headaches disappeared completely. However, some two years later, his symptoms returned. He admitted, when questioned, that he stopped following a gluten-free diet. When another blood test was taken, it showed the return of the anti-gliadin antibodies.

These results were enough to convince him that his headaches were caused by eating foods with gluten in them. He has since taken up a gluten-free diet that he has stuck with and has remained headache-free.

Another study disclosed that a patient had suffered from migraines for over ten years. The neurologists who were consulted could find no cure. The migraines became so intense he had to take an early retirement. By 2002 his three- times-a-week headaches had become constant. One particular month, he was headache-free for only three days. Migraine medications did not relieve this patient's pain.

The family doctor eventually suggested a gluten-free diet. The headaches gradually decreased, and after several months, he was 98% headache-free. Hooray! Gluten-free wins again!

Chapter 5

Gluten & Autism

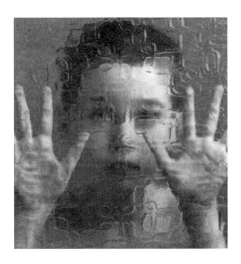

The subject of autism evokes a sensitive chord within me personally. I am the sibling of an autistic older brother. Defined as a neuro-developmental disorder that hinders communication and social interaction, autism usually develops by the time a child is three years old.

The sixties offered little to no solution for this enigmatic disability. I remember my parents taking my brother from one doctor to the next, trying to get answers as to, "what's wrong with Brian?"

Most of the medical physicians at the time had no clue. One offered to lobotomize Brian: my parents ran out of that doctor's office.

Fast forward decades later and there are still a lot of unanswered questions surrounding this ever-daunting disease. A look at the rise in numbers, tells a compelling story: The city of Atlanta, in 1996, compiled data from a mass observation system, which indicated that autism afflicted 3.4 per 1000 children ages three to 10 years old. That number increased to 6.7 per 1000 children three to 10 years old, according to a 1998 community study.

A report issued in May 2006 by the Center for Disease Control (CDC) suggests that at least 300,000 school-age children nationwide had autism in 2003 - 2004.

Parents tend to go to extreme measures when they find out their child is autistic, including drugs that control or neutralize the behavioral patterns.

The Autism Research Institute (ARI) collected information provided by over 23,700 parents who completed a questionnaire. ARI wanted to find which remedies were most successful in treating autism.

One of the most effective treatments was adhering to specific diet plans. This included removing gluten from the child's diet, with 65% of the parents reporting that their child got better.

No Talk, No way!

A nine-year-old boy was diagnosed with autism at the age of three. He had trouble focusing, never learned to speak, and had difficulty responding to communication. He finally started saying words voluntarily at the age of seven. When he was nine years old, his parents, with the encouragement of friends, put him on a gluten-free diet. Four months after his new eating plan started, the boy was potty trained, started reading, then began talking in long, sophisticated sentences, and was eventually able to interact with other children and adults.

Fit To Be Cried

A ten year old boy, who had been diagnosed at the age of four with autism, was displaying the typical behavioral characteristics: raging tantrums, kicking, biting himself, screaming, shoving, etc. His mother put him on a gluten-free diet on her own. The boy, within 3 weeks, began speaking in prolonged sentences. His temper tantrums decreased significantly, and over time he became much more friendly and lovable.

Autism is clearly defined. Celiac disease/gluten intolerance is well defined. Do they, however, relate to one another? That, my friends, is not well-defined.

Some exchanged research studies as to how they may be related are:

• Autism carries with it a higher prevalence of Celiac disease and gluten sensitivity. Some studies show that autistic kids have a three times higher rate of gluten disease than the general population. The question to ponder: Is this because people with autism are more likely to have Celiac disease? Or are people with Celiac disease more likely to be autistic?

• What if, at least in some cases, the autistic person actually has Celiac disease? Because the symptoms of Celiac disease and gluten sensitivity can mimic those of autism, are they, in fact, one and the same? It is completely understandable that a gluten-free diet would improve behaviors.

• Autism is separate from gluten disease, but similar in the fact that it responds well (sometimes in the case of autism) to a gluten-free diet.

• The main characteristic of gluten disease is malabsorption; could this result in a deficiency of important neurotransmitters in the brain, and thereby, create autistic behaviors?

• Reversely, could children who are diagnosed with gluten intolerance at a very early age and are subsequently put on a gluten-free diet *prevent* autistic behaviors from emerging by being gluten-free?

There definitely appears to be a connection between Celiac disease and autism, although the exact connection is not completely clear yet. It is well documented that autistic kids have gastrointestinal problems, and the commonness of gluten disease is higher in autistic patients than others. Due to poor digestion, the leaky gut syndrome that affects people with autism, causes large molecules, like gluten, to enter into the blood stream, setting off an autoimmune response.

The question is: which comes first? Do people with autism develop gluten disease more often because they have a leaky gut? Or does leaky gut syndrome allow gluten and other toxins into the body to cause autistic behaviors?

The correlation between gluten and behavior, expressly autism, is fascinating and worth exploring.

In addition to gluten-free dietary recommendations for autism, increasingly promising results have also been realized with the elimination of casein (pronounced KAY-seen) from the diet as well.

A Bit About Casein

Casein is the protein found in milk – not just cow's milk, but also in sheep and goat's milk. It is another protein strand that is difficult to digest and causes malabsorption.

A gluten-free/casein-free diet (aka GFCF) is currently one of the primary "alternative" treatments for autistic kids. The idea is that the sensitivities, or allergies these kids have to gluten and/or casein, causes a decline of mental capabilities that result in autistic behaviors. The removal of the offending proteins, gluten and casein, continue to show symptoms of poor focus, speech impediments, and impulsive behaviors were improved.

How do these significant occurrences happen?! Captain Opioid Strikes again!

Supporters of the GFCF diet have a definitive reason to why it works. It's called the *Opioid Excess Theory of*

Autism, first articulated by Kalle Reichelt in 1991.

The idea behind this theory is that those who are autistic metabolize gluten and casein differently from others. Gluten and casein are broken down into peptides called gliadinomorphin and casomorphine, respectively. A healthy process occurs within the body when these peptides are broken down further into essential amino acids – however, in autistic people they are not. The theory proclaims that instead, these peptides cross through the intestine into the bloodstream and ultimately, into the brain.

Because the chemical structures of gliadinomorphin and casomorphine are similar to that of morphine, a powerful opiate, they in turn have an addictive effect on the brain.

The high that is experienced is similar to that which an opium user would have. This could be why autistic kids exhibit various behaviors: finger flicking in front of their eyes, physically spinning around, head banging, a withdrawn demeanor, and being fascinated with parts of objects; like fixating on one part of a toy instead of the toy itself. Also, quite common of opiate users and autistic people is the distress they feel over small changes in their environment or routine.

Going gluten-free, can be very difficult for some people. Then, having to let go of the casein on top of it can seem like a virtual impossibility. I'm here to strongly encourage you: you can do it! For many people, the GF diet clears up a great amount of mental fog and allowed others to live a relatively pain-free life!

Most people who adhere to a dietary protocol are recommended to eliminate everything all at once, and then slowly introduce certain foods back into the diet. This procedure enables accurate tracking of how your body may react to certain foods.

Results on eating a gluten-free diet may vary. Some people see improvement within a week, some within a year's time frame; others may see no improvement at all. The reports for behavioral change differ as well. Some with autism have reported they are now able to sleep through the night. There are those who become more verbal and interactive, and others who report feelings completely normal as long as they adhere to their chosen diet.

There are yummy recipes in the back of the book for meals suggestions.

Chapter 6

What's Up Doc?

Then & Now: How Are Doctors Advising on Gluten?

Arteaeus of Cappadocia included a detailed description of the symptoms of gluten sensitivity in his writings as far back as 250 A.D.

In 1888 Dr. Samuel Gee of the Great Ormond Street Hospital for Children in the United Kingdom set out clinical accounts of the disease, and was quoted as saying, "If the patient can be cured at all, it must be by means of the diet."

Years later, in 1952 actually, Dr. Willem Karel Dicke, a Dutch pediatrician, identified wheat as the main culprit of many illnesses at that time. By the mid

1950s Dicke, along with a colleague, Professor Charlotte Anderson, and other researchers, working in Birmingham England, cornered gluten as *an offending protein*, and thereafter proclaimed the treatment for this condition was a gluten-free diet.

Throughout the 1950s, typical cases of Celiac disease were initially diagnosed by clinical observation of prevalent characteristics. Next was the invention of the endoscope; an instrument offering diagnosis by form of biopsy. Later, during the 1960s, improvements of testing procedures were implemented, including the development of serological screening for antigliadin IgA antibodies.

These tests enabled doctors to recognize the symptoms more readily, and observe the increase in incidents of this elusive disease.

Researchers in Europe began studying the widespread effects of gluten intolerance amongst the healthy population, as well as among people with various types of diseases such as osteoporosis, diabetes, and thyroid disease.

In 2004 Researcher William R. Treem wrote, "There has been an explosion in knowledge about Celiac disease over the last decade. Scientific studies of blood serum and other bodily fluids show that gluten intolerance is among the most common inherited diseases, with a worldwide prevalence of over 1%." This number has dramatically increased.

Today it is accepted that Celiac disease is a common disorder, not only in Europe (where it is most widespread) but also among of European ancestry, including those in North and South

America, Australia, North Africa, the
Middle East, and South Asia, where until
a few years ago it was considered rare.

The European food-processing
community has begun to adhere to the
demands for ready-made gluten-free
foods.

The Codex Alimentarius Commission,
along with the World Health
Organization, and the Food and
Agricultural Organization of the United
Nations, adopted the Codex Standard for
gluten-free foods so the public would
know if certain foods were really gluten-
free.

Other parts of the world have also
chosen to implement stricter standards
for gluten allowances with their food.
Canada's food and drug regulations, for
example, states: "No person shall label,
package, sell, or advertise food in a

manner likely to create an impression that it is gluten-free food unless the food does not contain wheat, including spelt and kamut, or oats, barley rye, triticale, or any part thereof."[3]

Australia and New Zealand are also on board with rigorous standards for gluten-free labeling. Their Food Standard code, 1.2.8, clauses 1 and 16, states that foods claiming to be gluten-free must not have detectable gluten, nor oats or cereals containing gluten that have been malted – a process where grains are sprouted from the seed by soaking them in water and then abruptly halted from germinating and dried with hot air.

Furthermore, food cannot be claimed to be "low gluten" unless it contains less than 20 mg. gluten, per 100 g of the food.

Finland, Sweden, and France are other countries that are supporting gluten-free labeling and menus as well.

How About the U.S.?

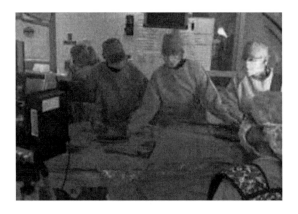

Why has the ailment of gluten and Celiac disease been hidden from the American Public for so long? It certainly can't be that the problem isn't devastating enough.

There is a strong possibility that the medical field may need more of an education in the field of gluten intolerance.

The curriculum for higher education programs to attain MD degrees are extremely rigorous and intense: Completion of four years of medical school, which include two years of classroom and laboratory study in anatomy, biochemistry, physiology, pharmacology, psychology, microbiology, pathology, medical ethics, and laws governing medicine. Such a challenging schedule is further compounded by, two years of working with patients under supervision; then usually three to eight years of internship and residency, when working in a specialized area of medicine.

However, despite its high level of achievement, students are neither equipped with academic or clinical instruction regarding gluten sensitivity.

It is to be strongly considered that the most significant research to impact the future of gluten is nutrition. Though medical science acknowledges that nutrition is inherent in neutralizing chronic diseases, higher education has been slow to integrate a viable nutrition component into their curriculum. Yet research continues to reveal the correlation of nutrition and gluten sensitivity.

Results of a survey published in 2004 by *Today's Dietician* revealed the ranking of nutrition taught in medical schools:

- Only 40% of all medical and osteopathic schools provide a separate required course requirement in nutrition.

- For schools that do require the study of nutrition, the average number of credit hours was only 2.5, with a range of 1 – 10 credits.

- Only 13 % of schools offer nutrition as an elective course.
- Roughly 24 % of colleges integrate nutrition into other courses.
- Elective courses of 2 credit hours attract only 25% of medical students.
- 23% of schools do not offer nutrition instruction at all.

With only marginal information regarding gluten intolerance is disclosed to medical students (mostly through a rotation in gastrointestinal medicine) along with the lack of a nutrition element in medical education, it's not surprising that symptoms aren't recognized and linked to gluten intolerance.

Hence, family physicians need to be familiar with the diagnosis and management of gluten sensitive diseases.[5]

The family physician or general practitioner is usually the first point of contact for patients. So, one would think the family physician would be prepared to use available research when confronted with signs of gluten sensitivity. However, as recently as 2005, surveys discovered that only 115 of Celiac patients were diagnosed by their primary care doctors. Further physician surveys revealed that only 35% of primary care doctors have ever diagnosed gluten intolerance!

An October 2010 issue of *Gastroenterology and Endoscopy* News quoted Dr. Peter Green as saying, "If a patient comes in, and he or she has gluten sensitivity, most doctors probably think, 'Where's the psychiatrist?' There is nothing taught about it and it's not currently measureable. Initially some of the Celiacs disease experts would roll their eyes claiming, 'We don't get into that. There's enough work to do to ascertain the diagnosis of Celiac disease, without the apparent allergy to gluten, it's even harder to define.' But the pressure is now on because the public is aware of it."

Is There Anybody Out There?

I mentioned in the introduction that medical practitioners are beginning to join together, to help heighten public awareness. These collaborations include the best of internal medicine, clinical nutrition, naturopathy, physical therapy, chiropractic, and more. The purpose is to work proactively together to resolve the individual's unique health problems and conditions.

A disturbing fact about the medical industry is the emphasis put on treating symptoms. How powerful it would be, if instead, every medical clinic in the world's goal was to find and fix the root cause of health problems?

Picture this: You are driving down the street and you hear your car making a strange sound. There is obviously a problem, so you take it to a mechanic. He tells you what to do.

He hands you a bag of earplugs and says, "Before you start your car, put these in your ears. This will make the noise go away. When you run out of ear plugs, come back and I'll give you some more."

This may sound absurd, but let's face it; this is often the kind of treatment most people receive from the medical industry. Or the doctor makes light of your problem, barely listens to what you're saying, or rushes you out of the office.

When dealing when gluten intolerance or any other debilitating disease, it is critical to be open to work with more than one health professional. Your body may need various kinds of treatments.

There are those who do not care to expend the effort to get well; some like the idea of swallowing a pill to temporarily feel better. If you do want to unravel why your body is creating certain symptoms, and you are willing to make some changes in your lifestyle, I want you to picture a new world that looks something like this:

Picture: Working with healthcare practitioners who are dedicated to solving your health problems, not just prescribing medication to block and mask symptoms, imagine medical professionals really listen to you and know the only way to truly help is by understanding what's going on inside the body. And imagine medical professionals who are aware and respect that no one knows that, better that you.

The first step for a new patient is to schedule a 30 minute complimentary consultation session. This meeting is to determine if the practitioners can help you; if so, how they would go about doing it. Not only do the healthcare professionals get a good history and feel for if they can help you, it gives you a feel for them, as well.

After the initial consultation, should all parties agree to move forward, schedule a more thorough examination. There, you could meet the medical director at that exam, as well as a physical therapist, and/or chiropractor; depending on the care you need. The point here is that you would be an active, informed participant in your own wellness process.

The doctors, afterwards, would get together to study your case in detail, and develop what will be the beginning of a treatment program to restore your body to good health. This may include one or several types of treatments, determined on a case-by-case basis.

The program would initially start with the basics, and become more refined, as the practitioners continue to indentify exactly what is causing your health problems. Having the expertise in many medical disciplines would offer a wide array of tests and treatments. There would be state-of-the-art laboratory testing, and an essential process of performing root cause analysis.

The emphasis on the wellness protocol would be placed on dietary changes, lifestyle management, home exercise programs, and nutritional supplements to name a few.

The chief mission is to use natural methods whenever possible. And when occasions to use medications are deemed necessary; which usually happens with the eradication of an infection, it would be done on a temporary basis, never as a sole treatment.

What if typical programs lasted 3 -4 months, and 90% of patients who followed their designed program experienced excellent changes in their health?

How awesome would it be if more medical programs like the one just described were more available? What if they become more widespread and continue to place emphasis on determining the root cause of illnesses, offering solutions that can heal in ways that naturally support the body's function?

I think we may just find out sooner than later. ☺

Roxanne McDonald

Chapter 7

Oh No! Not Fido & Frisky Too!

What may be viewed as *the* major flaw in the history of commercial pet foods is when the veterinary profession allowed the transition from corn to wheat based dry foods. This gross error took place in the mid 80s and opened up an unsavory can of worms, at least from our pet's point of view.

This sneaky, yet potentially very destructive condition, the very same gluten sensitivity we humans are suffering with, is prevalent among breeds of dogs and cats. Celiac researchers are now telling us that *all* who consume

today's processed gluten are likely to
become sensitive to it.

One definitive signal indicating your

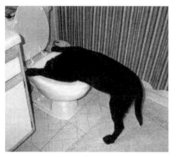

pet may very well be
suffering from
gluten intolerance
is the foul smell of
their passing gas.

Though, passing gas is normal in both
our pets and humans, if the condition
however, becomes chronic and the smell
reaches the stage where it's practically
unbearable, it's time to investigate the
matter.

How Do I Know Which Pet Food to Buy?

What does this mean when Fido
makes "happy" sounds while munching
on his scientifically formulated, well-
balanced food? This is the best quality,

right? The ill-fated truth of the matter is that pet food is not as scientifically formulated as most of us would like to believe or as the pet companies would have us believe. Purchasing the most expensive food, does not necessarily guarantee the highest nutritional levels.

Fido's food is typically made with convenience and the cost of manufacturing in mind. Science and nutrition may be secondary considerations. Though there are essential nutrients and vitamins added, and the food may look appealing enough, the main question is: Are these ingredients natural for the metabolism of your pet and are they readily available for body absorption? Herein lies the core of the matter.

Most cases of gluten intolerance show up in dogs and cats as skin or gastrointestinal disorders. These ultra sensitivity reactions are due to certain protein strands found in the diet. Such proteins as:

- Beef
- Dairy
- Eggs
- Lactose
- Other meat proteins
- Wheat
- Barley
- Rye
- Soy

Veterinary scientists have noted that gastrointestinal illnesses are the most common symptoms to look for.

A study of 55 cats with chronic intestinal problems showed that

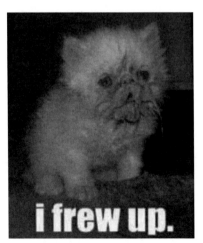

29 percent were food sensitive. Wheat, beef and corn gluten were names as the most common allergens.

Another study revealed that dogs had diarrhea and other gastrointestinal symptoms as a toxic reaction to gluten. The toxicity was proven by a biopsy that showed flattened villi.

In another case where 11 dogs with unfounded chronic colitis were treated for four months on a diet limited to chicken and rice (in other words, a gluten-free diet). Within one month, 60 percent of the dogs required no medication, or a reduced dosage of medication. Most conditions were completely cleared up after two months of being on the new diet.

It is very important to read the labels on the can or package of your pet's food. Also, bear in mind that just like with *people food*, pet food ingredients are listed in the order of volume.

A can of store brand dog food states the food within has, "no added preservatives, formulated for healthy skin and coat, highly digestible, soy free." The first five ingredients listed are: chicken, meat by-products, ground rice, wheat flour, and wheat gluten. These are its *top* ingredients. It is loaded with gluten. And so are most cat food.

Many informed people have taken their dogs off of commercial dog food, and now feed them home- cooked chicken, carrots, and rice. You can occasionally mix in other vegetables, and even fruit.

The results: no bloating, diarrhea, or super foul-smelling gas.

I have been recovering from the pangs of eating gluten for the past three years. I simply dismissed the constant gas, intestinal discomfort, and more recent joint aches (in my fingers in particular) as something I ate that disagreed with me. I wasn't too far off with the *something I ate* part. However, I had no idea that it was gluten in most of the things I was eating.

Hundreds of thousands of people are learning about this disease and changing their diets. Human beings are closely related to dogs and cats, genetically speaking, therefore we are susceptible to the same type of chronic diseases.

A universal solution for both two-legged and four-legged creatures is to take the time to prepare the food yourself. You will be happy, and your pet will be happy. Now when you open up the windows, it will be to let the sunshine in and circulate the fresh air that's already in the room. ☺

Roxanne McDonald

Chapter 8

Free At Last!

Gluten-free Living – Be In Charge and Live Affordably

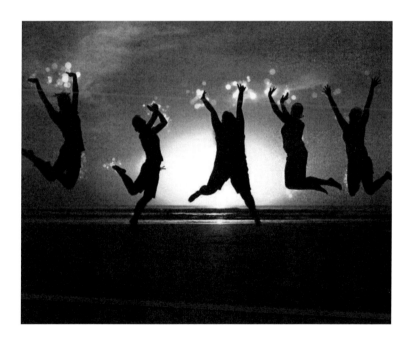

You may be wondering, where and how am I going to shop, living in this gluten-free world? Great question!

Those who have been eating gluten-free for a long while and dreamt of a marketplace that supported their lifestyle, are now reveling in the reality of shopping at gluten-free stores.

Other resources include stores filled with gluten-free foods, books about living a gluten-free lifestyle; cookbooks and other vital resources. The great news is, these businesses are actually thriving!

One of the most common complaints expressed about eating gluten-free is that it's more expensive. It doesn't need to be. Yes, gluten-free cookies are smaller and twice the price of regular cookies, and no one could argue that regular bread is typically less than half the cost of a loaf of gluten-free bread, but there are ways to save a substantial amount of money while enjoying a gluten-free lifestyle. There is no need to take out a second loan on your home. ☺

Most of the "extra expense" of eating a gluten-free diet is spent on the high cost of specialty items. I recognize your need to have some specialty items on hand, like cake for example. It would be really awkward trying to stick a candle into little Emily's rice cracker for her birthday.

Should you find that you are spending more money than your budget can stand eating gluten free, take a look at what types, and how many specialty items you are buying. Breads, crackers, cookies, cakes, pizza, pretzels, and donuts; they're pricey, and you don't need them. You can substitute store-bought chips for a fraction of the cost of gluten-free pretzels or kale chips. The reality is, most of the specialty items aren't good for you anyway – they're high calorie, high-glycemic-index foods that will quickly raise your blood sugar. These items will definitely put a burden on the budget.

Where Else You Can Shop?

Farmer's markets, found on a corner near you, are popping up everywhere offering fresh produce, eggs, meat, fish honey, nuts, and other inherently gluten-free items, usually at prices far below those of retailers. The foods sold there are naturally ripe. Organic is the rule rather than the exception, and the generous samples that sellers pass out are enough to count as a meal.

You can also feel good knowing that you're supporting your local farmers and the environment. The food is usually grown without pesticides, and not having to ship long distances, saves on energy and gas.

Some of the ethnic markets are truly worth visiting for gluten-free food:

- Asian: the more authentic the better.
- Thai and Indian aisles for their sauces, rice wraps, the list goes on.
- Mexican food also uses gluten-free ingredients in their cooking.
- Mediterranean diets are highly recommended for vegan and gluten free eating.

You may explore foods from other cultures without leaving the country and experience the fun and variety of eating gluten-free.

Navigating Through Stores

You have probably thought that grocery shopping was just a matter of wheeling the cart up and down the aisles, right? And you most likely have felt that you were in control of your purchases.

Psychologists hired by the grocery industry have, for decades now, been researching ways to get people to spend more money. They actually come up with subtle and subliminal ways to *cast a spell* on people. These poor souls fall prey to strategically placed temptations, scattered throughout the store like booby traps. I've been there!

Here's a suggestion to take control of your shopping again: carry a list of safe & unsafe ingredients for label reading when you go shopping. Check out Celiac.com for more details.

Billions of retail-funded dollars are spent on these high-powered grocery store psychologists, and the discoveries are somewhat alarming. Let's face it; many shoppers are impulsive. The stores take advantage of your impulsivity, by orchestrating emotionally-based purchases.

"Planned impulsivity", as it were, may seem like a contradiction in terms, but there is a precise strategy to what the stores are devising when they design everything from where to plant items to what music to play in the background.

We've all fallen for the marketing ploy: You're at the store for only a few items. You walk in carrying the smaller hand basket, and you walk out with a cartload of things you really didn't want. It's the flashing coupon dispensers, the in aisle displays, the free samples, and heavily-loaded spreads at the end of each aisle; all a by-product of the psychologist's assignment. And let's not forget the fact that kids are a direct target, as they tend to influence impulsive purchases.

Unfortunately, seldom are these subconsciously influenced purchases directing you towards healthy food, much less gluten-free food. when the temptation to devour gluten products seems overbearing, be extra cautious about how stores can cast a hypnotic allure over you - one that coaxes you to fill your basket with foods you don't need and that are unhealthy for you.

It's really about developing healthy shopping habits. Here are some thoughts to keep in mind that will save time and money when you shop:

• Don't shop hungry. You are quite vulnerable when hungry to be subjected to impulsive buying.

• Bring a list. Pre planning before shopping can help you to focus on the gluten-free and healthy foods you need.

• Consider co-ops . If you happen to have one nearby, they're a great way to save money. Cooperatives are made up of groups of people who buy food in bulk, and then offer the food to others to buy. Typically, anyone can become a member for a small charge; nonmembers can buy too, but usually for a surcharge. The focus is usually on healthy foods.

• Join membership clubs. Membership clubs are, as a rule, big warehouse-type stores. Sam's Club, one of the world's largest (Sam's Club) is now carrying a large selection of gluten-free products. These stores are known for carrying products in bulk.

• Use coupons, fliers, rebates, and frequent-shopper programs. You can save hundreds of dollars each year by using coupons. Even if you're not thrilled with the chore of coupon clipping, try to find a few to use each week, in your local newspaper or online and check the circulars that are in front of the store as well. They advertise specials for the week and they're usually for produce, which is gluten-free.

• Take the comparison challenge. Always look at the unit price of a product, not just the package price. Stores list unit prices on the price tags on the grocery shelves. The package price tells you only the cost of the entire item, whereas the unit price shows the cost per pound, ounce, and so forth. This enables you to compare apples to apples instead of just comparing one price to another. A calculator would certainly come in handy for the most accurate calculations.

• Keep your eye on the scanner. Meaning you may have to forsake the tabloids that are *ragging* on some celeb for giving birth to twin orangutans, or how to fog up a mirror and lose ten pounds at the same time. However, watching to make sure the scanner rings up the correct price is more important. Stores do make mistakes, and many times not in your favor.

• It's also very important to bear in mind that though an item is tagged gluten free, it may have other ingredients that are just as harmful or worse. The various starches that are used to provide a level of consistency for certain products are laden with high fructose sugars, which will cause massive blood spiking in the body. The process of what we ingest and how it breaks down (metabolizes) in our body is ultimately critical to our overall health.

• If possible, don't shop with your kids – We love them beyond measure, don't we? But they are the number one enemy when trying not to shop impulsively. They are primary targets of sales gimmicks. Observe how the sugary cereals are located right at the eye level of an impressionable five-year-old. Grocery stores are counting on your kids to lure you into impulsive purchases of high-profit margin treats like cereals and snack foods.

The ultimate goal here is to equip yourself with as much information as possible, to live and enjoy living a healthy, gluten–free lifestyle. No pills. No shots. No surgical solution. The only way to treat gluten sensitivity is to eliminate gluten from your diet.

You have the power of choice! Use it & live your *epic health epic health now*!

Roxanne McDonald

Bonus Chapter

The 8 Steps to Staying Gluten-free

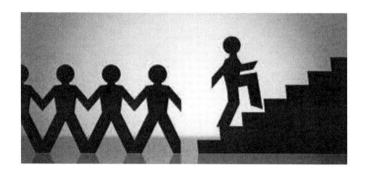

1. Get checked for gluten intolerance if you have any of the ailments previously discussed in this book.

2. Realize you have no power over gluten and to continue to eat foods that contain gluten would be insane.

3. Admit to yourself and someone else (aside from your Higher Power, though it is highly recommended you do admit it to your HP as well) that you do not have

control over gluten, and your passing gas has become unmanageable.

4. Write down your feelings instead, when you experience an attack of the "craves" and are prepared to lie and cheat and steal to get a gluten fix.

5. Begin to associate and become friends with other gluten-free members of your community.

6. Gather recipes, patronize stores with gluten-free sections, and visit restaurants that also support gluten-free lifestyles -- they are out there!

7. Continue to take personal inventory of your eating habits. Your body will appreciate it. And if you have a slip, love yourself, and get back on the gluten-free bandwagon.

8. It is likely you may have a spiritual awakening from living a gluten-free life; either way you will feel so much better

you'll want to share your experience, strength and health with others, and join in the quest for epic health now!

Roxanne McDonald

DELICIOUS GLUTEN-FREE RECIPES:

Desserts

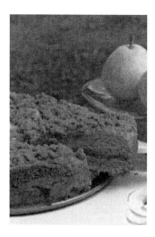

Gluten-free and Vegan Pear Coffee Cake

This stunning coffee cake uses coconut based vanilla bean ice cream and pear puree. The ice cream adds protein and the pear puree, like applesauce, contains pectin which tenderizes the cake.

- 1 cup sugar: coconut sugar, raw cane sugar or certified beet sugar
- 1 ½ cups almond or coconut gluten-free all purpose flour blend
- ½ cup sorghum flour
- 1 tablespoon of agar*
- ½ teaspoon Celtic or Himalayan sea salt*
- 2 teaspoons baking powder
- 1 teaspoon baking soda
- 1½ cups coconut based vanilla bean ice cream.
- 6 tablespoons organic coconut oil

- 4 tablespoons pureed baby pear puree or unsweetened   applesauce
- ½ cup peeled and chopped ripe organic Bartlett, Bosc or red pears.
- Crumble Topping (below)

Preheat the oven to 325°F and lightly oil a 9-inch springform pan.

Combine the sugar, flour blend, sorghum flour, salt, baking powder, and baking soda in a large bowl. Set aside.

Combine the coconut – based ice cream, organic coconut oil, and pear puree in a mixing bowl and beat until smooth. Add the dry ingredients and beat until smooth. Fold in chopped fruit.

Spoon half the batter over the bottom of the prepared pan and smooth to the edges of the pan. Cover with half of the crumb mixture. Spoon the remaining batter over the crumb topping and smooth to the edges. Sprinkle the remaining topping over the top.

Bake 50 to 55 minutes, until cake tester comes out clean and center springs back when gently touched. Cool 10 minutes in the pan. Remove the rim of the pan and cool completely on a wire rack. Serve.

*If your all-purpose blend contains salt and agar, omit the salt and reduce the agar to ½ teaspoon.

Crumble Topping ½ cup rice flour ½ cup packed coconut sugar 2 teaspoons ground cinnamon ¼ teaspoon ground allspice 1/8 teaspoon ground cloves ¼ teaspoon salt 4 tablespoons non-dairy buttery spread, at room temperature

Combine the flour, coconut sugar, cinnamon, allspice, cloves, and salt in a large bowl. Mix well. Add the butter and use fingertips or a fork to mix just until crumbly.

This can be made ahead and stored in the refrigerator for up to 2 weeks.

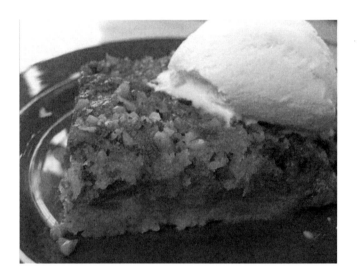

Apple Walnut Cobbler (Wheat Free)

Pure maple syrup brushed on the warm cobbler adds color and shine to the other-wise pale topping. And don't save this excellent cobbler for wheat-sensitive people only; everyone will like it.

Serves: 6 to 8

Filling:

- 5 tablespoons pure maple syrup
- 1 tablespoon arrowroot
- 2 teaspoons fresh lemon juice
- Dash salt
- 5 cups apple slices, unpeeled or peeled (about 2 pounds)

- 1/2 cup walnuts, chopped, toasted, and cooled

Topping:

- 1/2 cup oat flour (see note)
- 2 tablespoons coconut sugar
- 3/4 teaspoon ground Ceylon cinnamon
- 3/4 teaspoon baking powder
- 1/4 teaspoon baking soda
- Dash salt
- 3 tablespoons olive oil
- 3 tablespoons organic pure maple syrup
- 6 tablespoons almond or hempseed milk
- 1 teaspoon pure vanilla extract

Position a rack in the middle of the oven and preheat to 350 degrees. Lightly oil a 9-inch deep-dish pie pan or 2-quart baking dish.

To make the filling, mix the maple syrup and arrowroot in a large bowl until well blended. Add the lemon juice and salt. Add the apples and toss until coated.

To make the topping, combine the oat flour, dark whole cane sugar, cinnamon, baking powder, baking soda, and salt in a medium bowl, and stir to mix.

Combine the oil with 1 tablespoon of the maple syrup in a small bowl. Add the soymilk and vanilla, and mix until well blended. Pour into the oat mixture and mix until a soft dough forms.

Spoon the topping over the fruit and bake for 25 to 35 minutes, until the topping is firm and the fruit is bubbling. Remove from the oven and brush with the remaining 2 tablespoons maple syrup. Cool about 5 minutes and serve warm from the baking dish.

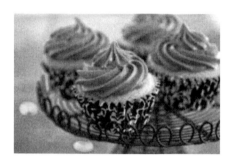

Banana- Scented Vanilla Cakes or Cupcakes

This cake has just a light banana flavor combined with fragrant vanilla. The banana helps add stability and moistness so don't leave it out to make a vanilla-only cake. It is such a subtle flavor that is most lovely, and the cake is fluffy and moist, perfect for any special occasion.

Makes 2 round cake layers

- 1 cup millet flour
- ¾ cup almond flour (see note)
- ¼ cup arrowroot powder
- 1 teaspoon agar powder
- ½ teaspoon baking soda
- 2 teaspoons baking powder
- 1 coconut sugar
- ½ teaspoon (scant) Celtic sea salt
- 1 cup + 2 tablespoons of almond or hemp milk
  ¾ cup pureed ripe banana (1½ to 2 small bananas, or 1½ medium-to large)

115

- 1 tablespoon apple cider vinegar
- 1½ teaspoons pure vanilla extract
- ⅓ cup organic coconut oil

Cooked Chocolate Frosting (recipe follows)

Preheat the oven to 350°F. Lightly oil two 8-inch round cake pans and line the bottom of each with parchment paper, if you desire.

In a large bowl, combine the flours, agar; sift in the baking powder and baking soda; then add the coconut sugar and Celtic sea salt. Mix well.

In another bowl, stir the nondairy milk and banana together, and then add the vinegar, extract, and oil. Add the wet mixture to the dry, and stir until incorporated.

Pour the batter evenly into the prepared pans. Bake for 27 to 30 minutes, or until a toothpick inserted in the center of each comes out clean.

Remove from the oven and let cool in the pans on a cooling rack.

Note: Oat flour is available in natural foods stores and some supermarkets, but if you have rolled oats on hand, you can grind them into flour in a blender or food processor, a few cups at a time. To make 1 cup of oat flour, start with 1 1/4 cups rolled oats. Store the flour in a zip-lock plastic bag or tightly closed container in the freezer for up to two months. This cake has just a light banana flavor combined with fragrant vanilla. The banana helps add stability and moistness so don't leave it out to make a vanilla-only cake. It is such a subtle flavor that is most lovely, and the cake is fluffy and moist, perfect for any special occasion.

Use an immersion blender or mini processor to puree the banana.

This cake takes a little longer to set up than some other cake recipes. Just have patience, and watch until the layers become lightly golden around the edges and the centers are no longer dull and sticky looking (and test with a toothpick)!

Cupcake variation: To adapt this cake to cupcakes, line twenty to twenty-two compartments of a muffin tin and fill about halfway with the batter. Bake in a preheated 350°F oven for 22 to 24 minutes (test with a toothpick).

Substitutions: You can use almond flour, brown rice flour, or a combination of both. Note that white rice flour gives a slightly lighter cake texture, and brown rice flour can impart a subtle aftertaste. For taste and texture, using all or some of white rice flour is preferred.

Cooked Chocolate Frosting

Makes enough frosting for one 2-layer cake

- 5 tablespoons millet (for gluten-free), almond flour, or coconut flour.
  or spelt flour (see note)
- 1¼ cups natural powdered sugar, sifted if lumpy

- 3 tablespoons unsweetened cacao powder
- ½ teaspoon sea salt
- ¼ or ½ teaspoon agar powder (use ¼ teaspoon for fruit flour
  or spelt flour, ½ teaspoon for millet)
- 1 cup + 2 tablespoons chocolate nondairy milk (see note)
- ½ cup organic extra-virgin coconut oil, at room temperature

In a saucepan over medium heat, whisk the flour with the sugar, cocoa, salt, and agar. Gradually whisk in the milk. Cook, stirring frequently with a whisk at first, and then whisk almost constantly as the mixture thickens (take care that the mixture doesn't thicken on the bottom of the pan and clump; lower the heat to medium-low, if necessary).

Transfer to a stand mixer fitted with the paddle attachment. Mix on high speed for about 5 minutes, until the mixture has started to cool down. Add the coconut oil and beat for another few minutes, until the mixture is cool and creamy. At this point, you can either frost your cake or chill the frosting to whip up even fluffier.

To do so, refrigerate the mixer bowl of frosting until chilled (1 to 1½ hours). Then, instead of using the paddle attachment, affix the wire whisk attachment. Begin mixing slowly and then bring up to the fastest speed for a minute or two, until the frosting becomes lighter in color and fluffier. (If it doesn't, the frosting might need more chilling. Return the bowl to fridge for another 30 minutes to an hour. Then whip at high speed again.)

Frost the cake or refrigerate the whipped mixture.

Note: When using millet flour, because it is gluten-free, it is helpful to use extra agar to help stabilize the frosting.

Roxanne McDonald

Entrees

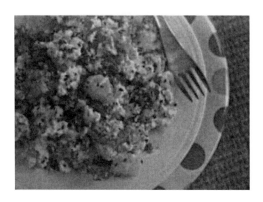

Creamy Chick pea Scramble With Kale and Pumpkin

or Butternut Squash

This recipe proves that you don't need a ton of ingredients to create a flavorful recipe. This delicious and very pretty tofu scramble features pumpkin or butternut squash and kale, making it perfect seasonal fare for a super-quick dinner (providing that your pumpkin or squash is pre-baked; brunch, or even a hearty breakfast.

Serves: 4 or more

- 12 to 16 ounces softened chick peas
- 1 tablespoon coconut oil, preferably organic
- 1/4 to 1/2 cup vegetable broth or stock, as needed
- 5 leaves kale, midrib removed, coarsely chopped
- 2 cups cooked pumpkin or butternut squash, cut into 1-inch   cubes

- 1 recipe
- Sprinkle of sesame seasoning (you can also use Eden Shake, or   use gomashio)

Let chick peas soak in water over night. Then boil chick peas under medium high heat for 2 hours or until soft.

Crumble the chick peas into bite-sized pieces, or cut into small cubes. Heat the oil in a large nonstick frying pan over medium-high heat and add chick peas. Brown on all sides until lightly golden.

Add the broth and kale and cook for another minute or two, until the kale begins to wilt a bit. Add the pumpkin and dressing and gently stir to coat everything. Lower heat to simmer, cover, and allow to heat through, stirring once or twice, about 10 minutes. Serve garnished with sesame seasoning.

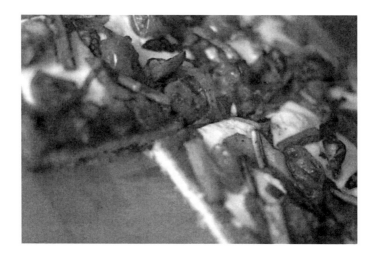

Parade Pan Pizza

Pizza is a fun way to eat vegetables, however, tasty gluten-free crusts can be difficult to find. This crust is based on whole-grain brown rice, which you can find in any grocery store. Some toppings are suggested but any will do. Experiment!

- 1cup uncooked brown rice
- 3 cups grated cashew cheese
- 1 egg, slightly beaten
- 2 cups tomato sauce
- 1 teaspoon garlic powder
- 1 teaspoon dried oregano
- 1teaspoon dried basil
- 1 small onion, chopped
- 1 red bell pepper, diced
- 1 green bell pepper, diced
- ½ cup mushrooms, sliced
- ½ cup grated cashew cheese Makes 1 pizza
- ¼ cup of spring water

- 1 teaspoon of probiotic powder or emptied capsule
- 2 tbsp nutritional yeast flakes, powdered or crushed up between your fingers
- 2 tsp onion powder
- 1 tsp garlic powder
- 1 tbsp lemon juice
- 1 - 2 tsp crystal salt

Cashew Cheese Preparation:

1 pound of cashews soaked & rinsed. Soak 4 – 6 hours
Next, blend cashews, the water & the probiotic powder using the tamper stick to help the mixture blend into a smooth consistency.

Transfer the mix into a nut milk bag and squeeze out some of the excess water, this will help yield a firmer cheese.

Using a steamer basket with a pot underneath, place the cheese (still in the nut milk bag) into the strainer and place a weight on top of it. A 2 liter jar filled with water works well.

Cover with a kitchen towel and place it into a warm place for 12 -24 hours to ferment. Airing in the cupboard or over a dehydrator (while it's running) are great places,

After the appointed time, the mixture should have a pungent smell & a slightly sour taste.

Next, transfer to a mixing bowl and now it's time to season the cheese so it tastes like cheese.

Add the nutritional yeast flakes, onion powder, garlic powder, lemon juice & crystal salt and mix well to combine. Set aside, briefly.

Preheat oven to 425 degrees F. Lightly oil (Virgin olive or raw coconut) a 12" round or 11" x 19 rectangular pizza pan or an 11" x 13" shallow baking dish.

Prepare the rice as directed on package. Immediately after the rice is cooked, ad 1 cup of the cheese mixture. Stir well to blend all ingredients and melt the cheese. Spread the rice mixture evenly on greased pan. Bake 15 minutes only, and remove crust from oven.
Spread tomato sauce evenly over crust, and sprinkle with garlic powder, oregano, and basil. Arrange onion, peppers, and mushrooms evenly over the top. Top with the remaining cashew cheese. Return pizza to oven, and bake an additional 5 minutes or until the sauce is hot and the cheese is melted. Let the pizza sit for 5 minutes before cutting.

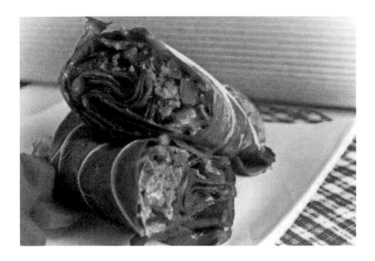

Raw Walnut Burritos

This dandy treat will have folks talking for a long time after they experience the tantalizing tastes that will linger on their palates. It's raw "at its' best". You'll be forever dubbed a master chef, and they will come back for more!

Raw Walnut Meat Ingredients:
- ½ cup walnuts (soaked for 1 hour)
- 1 pinch cumin
- 1 pinch coriander
- Splash of tamari

Process:
Blend all the ingredients in the food processor or blender for a minute or so.

Raw Salsa Ingredients
- 1 small organic red onion
- 1 pint organic cherry tomatoes
- 1 small organic green pepper

- 1 handful cilantro
- 1 tbsp cumin
- 1 lime (juiced)
- Cayenne to taste
- Sea salt to taste

Process:
Put food in food processor or blender, and pulse for 10 -15 times.

Mexican Rice Ingredients:
- ¼ head of cabbage, shredded
- ½ small sweet onion
- 2 tbsp sun-dried tomato powder
- ½ tbsp extra-virgin olive oil
- ½ tsp salt
- ¼ tsp chili power or more to liking
- ¼ tsp cumin
- ½ clove garlic
- ½ ripe tomato, diced

Process:

Place cabbage in food processor fitted with an 's' blade and pulse until rice like texture. Transfer to large bowl and add onion, sun-dried tomato powder, oil, salt, chili powder, cumin, onion powder, garlic, and tomato, toss gently. You can warm it in a dehydrator set at 125 degrees for 30 minutes – to 2 hours, if you like.

Finally…the Raw Burrito Ingredients
- 2 collard leaves
- 1 cup lettuce
- 1 small handful of cilantro

- ½ cup chopped avocado
- (And anything else you want inside)

Process:
De-stem the collards. Cut up the lettuce, cilantro and avocado. Fill the collards with all the good stuff above and wrap them up like a burrito.
Next…Chow Down!!

Salad Dressings

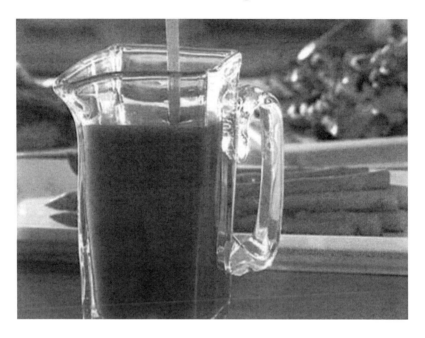

Put these scrumptious dressings on your favorite fresh organic salads

Creamy Basil Pesto Salad Dressing

Ingredients:

- 1 cup basil
- 1/3 cup pine nuts
- ¼ cup olive oil
- 5 cloves garlic
- ½ piece of lemon (peeled)
- ½ of lemon (juice)
- ½ tbsp raw honey
- Water to consistency

Process:
Blend and then make your salad.

Dressing Ingredients:
- 2 tbsp olive oil
- 2 tbsp mustard
- 1tbsp water
- 2 tsp apple cider vinegar
- 1pinch sea salt
- 1 pinch black pepper

Process:
Mix with other ingredients and pour over salad.

You can also use kelp noodles with this meal. Kelp noodles are a great pasta alternative and are delicious in salad. Rinse kelp noodles really well, then soak then for 15-20 minutes. You can purchase these are most health food stores.

Raw Tahini Sauce Ingredients:
- 4 Tbsp water
- 3 tbsp tamari
- 3-4 tsp raw tahini (more if you want it thicker)
- 2 tsp raw olive oil (or sesame oil)
- 1 tbsp honey (for vegan, use pure maple syrup
- 1 tbsp ginger
- 1 clove garlic
- 1 tbsp lemon juice
- 1 pinch cumin
- 1 pinch sea salt

Process: Blend

"Dragon Green Salad Dressing"

Recipe By: Truth Calkins
Taste: Spicy, hot, salty, tangy, with a touch of sweet
Beneficial For: Candida, Cleansing, Detoxification, and Increasing Circulation
Suggested Usage: Add on top of fish, cooked veggies, quinoa, salad, or just about anything else!
Shelf-Life/Storage: Store in a glass jar in the refrigerator. Will last a very long time. If it separates, shake before pouring.

Ingredients:
- Large bunch of Cilantro
- 1 Organic Yellow Onion
- 1 Organic Jalapeno Pepper
- Oshsawa Organic Tamari

Process:

Cut Jalapeno pepper, Cilantro, and Onion into chunks. Add to blender in that order.
Add Tamari, Flaxseed Oil, Olive Oil, and Apple Cider Vinegar to the blender in that order.
Add Marine Phytoplankton, Ashitaba, and Chlorella Powder to the blender in that order.
Add Super Ionic and Stevia to the blender in that order.
Blend well and enjoy!

Roxanne McDonald

Smoothies

It may sound weird, but be open to following these simple directions on how to eat a smoothie. You can use a straw, a spoon, sip from a glass; either way, be sure to chew it a bit before you swallow. This will start your saliva glands producing saliva to aid with digestion. Be sure to eat your smoothie like it's a sit down meal. So eat it within 20 minutes for the best digestion.

Mango Tango Ingredients:

- 4 mangoes
- 5 bananas
- 4 cups of spinach
- 8 stalks of celery
- Meat from 1 young coconut of ¼ cup pre-soaked flax seed.

Process: Blend. Drink half and save the rest for lunch

Sweet Kale Ingredients:

- 4 bananas
- 5 Bosc pears
- 1 cup raspberries
- 4 kale leaves
- ½ lemon
- ¼ cup flax seed

Optional:
Chlorella, B-Flax-D, Green Powder

Process:
Blend. Drink half and save the other half for lunch

Each one of us has different caloric needs so if you need more, make more!

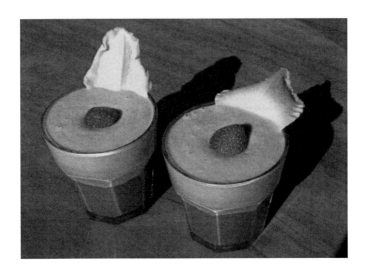

Chocolate Super Food Smoothie Recipe: "Chocolate Vanilla Bean Dream"
Recipe By: David Wolfe

Ingredients:
- 3 TBSP Cacao Powder

- 1 TBSP Maca Powder

- 1 tsp Ceylon Cinnamon
- 1 TBSP Cacao Nibs

- 3-4 TBSP liquid Coconut Oil

- 1-2 TBSP Cashews

- 1-3 TBSP Noniland Honey

- 1 TBSP Hemp Seed

- 1/2 tsp or less of Sea Salt

- 1/2 tsp or less of Ginger
- 1/2 tsp or less of Cayenne
- 1 tsp Ground Vanilla

- 6 inch chunk Aloe Vera Gel, filleted and skinned
- 1 tsp - 1 TBSP Medicinal Mushroom Mycelium (24 Mushroom   Blend)
- 5-6 cups Liquid Base: Spring water, any tea, coconut water
- 1 squirt Crystal Energy

Directions:
Add Dry Ingredients to the Blender.
Add Wet Ingredients to the Blender.
Blend and Enjoy!

Roxanne McDonald

References

1. Living Gluten- Free for Dummies. Danna Korn.

2. St. Bartholomew's Hospital Report, Article, "On the Coeliac Affection," 1888.

3. Everyday Health Magazine.

4. The Annals of Medicine Magazine, 2010.

5. The Gluten-free Nutrition Guide. Tricia Thompson, M.S., RD.

6. The Gluten Connection. Shari Lieberman, PhD, CNS, FACN, with Linda Segall.

7. Archives of Internal Medicine Magazine, (2003).

8. Gastroenterology and Endoscopy News, (2010).

9. European Food Safety Authority. Opinion of the Scientific Panel on Dietetic

Products, Nutrition and Allergies on a request from the Commission related to a notification from AAC on wheat-based glucose syrups including dextrose. EFSA Journal 126, (2004).

10.   Celiac Sprue Association, CSA Recognition Seal Program. CSA website, csaCeliacs.org/CSA SealofRecognition.php

About the Author

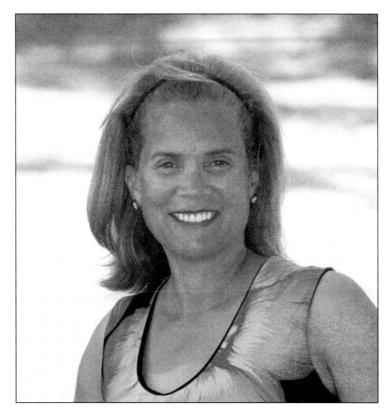

Roxanne McDonald is a Body Mind Institute certified nutrition expert, a writer, a social entrepreneur, public speaker, and author of her first book: Breaking up with Gluten- Ways to Clean out Your Gut and Save Your Butt!

A graduate of California State University, Los Angeles, Roxanne received a Bachelor of Arts degree in English Literature, and also minored in economics. She garnered a successful 20 year stint with Corporate America as a sales and marketing executive in the telecommunications, software and real estate industries. Initially, after graduation from college, as her quest for adventure would have its way, Roxanne chose to take to the high seas and became a merchant marine. "The opportunity to travel the world working on various cargo and passenger ships, proved to be an invaluable experience beyond measure."

Roxanne's inclination and sheer enjoyment for eating a variety of foods was enhanced by her travels, where she readily conceded to being a bona fide foodie. Years went by and the pleasure of the palate seemed to know no bounds, until one day Roxanne found herself at an outdoor jazz event where many vendors were touting their wares at their respective booths. Upon venturing into a wellness practitioner's place of business, followed by a brief blood and saliva test, Roxanne was told she had an allergy to wheat. "Whatever that means" is how that bit of information was processed at the time. And her eating habits continued along their eager path.

As more time passed, Roxanne noticed she was having chronic difficulty with digestion and increased gastric issues. A routine check up at the doctor's office was met with diagnoses of diverticulitis and colitis. Basically, the colon and intestinal tract where inflamed and wreaking havoc inside her body. She began a journey to learn more about these kinds of ailments in relation to her eating habits and what could be done to bring about relief. The information acquired about gluten intolerance and celiac disease was an absolute wake-up call as research shed light on the origin of these illnesses and their direct connection with eating certain grains as well as other product consumption.

Roxanne has since incorporated new eating habits with emphasis on an organic, plant-based, raw food lifestyle. "I still love to eat warm food, just not as often and not as hot as I used to eat it; over cooking vegetables takes the nutrients right out of them. We want to maintain a level of crunch to the texture."

Since embracing a healthier lifestyle around eating and having a better understanding with her relationship with food, the colitis and diverticulitis conditions have been eliminated. And the joint pains that were beginning to surface have disappeared as well. Roxanne has repeatedly proven to herself that there is a direct correlation with what she eats and how it affects the health of her body. The aforementioned research continues to expand, including proven case studies and working with others with similar results.

Get the Real Skinny on Gluten –Free Living covers graphic detail on history of gluten and the consequences of ingesting foods and putting other substances, e.g., makeup on your skin that contain gluten. Most importantly, the book reveals ways that you can displace and eventually replace toxic substances with organic (derived from living organisms – we want food to be alive, not dead) healthier ways of living that your body, mind and spirit will love!

Roxanne was born the youngest of three children. The influence from her minister father and educator mother is tremendous and consciously integrated into her presentations. She offers a delivery style of "edutainment" to her audience, and continues to encourage folks to actively check in with their "heart-spirit" and trust how it feels. "There is no better time that the present to live your epic health now!"

Roxanne McDonald